ACCUTANE

The ultimate guide ⌐   ⧸ to use Accutane powerful medication to treat severe acne that has not responded to other treatments.

Dr. Joseph Smith

Table of Contents

CHAPTER 1

WHAT IS THE PURPOSE OF ACCUTANE?

Isotretinoin is the key component of the medication Accutane. Acne is treated with Accutane.

Accutane is a member of a class of drugs known as retinoids that are related to vitamin A.

Retinoids function by lowering the quantity of sebum (an oily material produced by skin glands), lowering bacterial growth and irritation, and unclogging blocked pores.

Acne is treated with several different kinds of medications. For more severe situations, Accutane is prescribed.

Yet, there's a chance that your doctor gave you Accutane for a different reason.

If you have any inquiries regarding why Accutane has been recommended for you, speak with your doctor.

Just a doctor's prescription is required to get this medication. There is no addiction to Accutane

PRIOR TO BEGINNING ACCUTANE

When you shouldn't accept it

If any of the following apply to you: 1. you are pregnant or intend to become pregnant within the next month, do not use Accutane.

If you become pregnant while using Accutane, your chances of having a severely malformed child are quite high. Effective contraception must be used for a month before to, during, and after therapy.

2. You are nursing.

Breastfeeding must end before therapy can start. If you are on Accutane, stop breastfeeding.

3. any of the substances specified at the end of this leaflet, vitamin A, other retinoids, or Accutane has caused an adverse response in the past.

4. You are taking antibiotics with tetracycline.

5. You have a serious liver condition.

6. Your blood fat levels (cholesterol and triglycerides) are very high.

7. You suffer from A hypervitaminosis

This illness is brought on by consuming too much vitamin A.

8. There are rips in the packing or other evidence of tampering

9. The pack's printed expiration date (EXP) has past.

It may not function as effectively if you take this medication after the expiration date has past.

Contact your doctor if you're unsure if you should begin taking Accutane.

Children should not be given Accutane.

When given to children before puberty, roccutane may cause a slowdown in growth. Accutane should not be administered to children less than 12 years of age.

BEFORE YOU BEGIN TAKING IT

If you: 1. have any allergies to any other medications, foods, preservatives, or colours, you must inform your doctor.

Soya oil, which is a component of Accutane capsules and may include quantities of arachidic acid (a component of peanut oil)

2. You currently have or have ever had any other health difficulties or problems, such as diabetes or a family history of the disease.

depression

liver illness

renal illness

hormone condition caused by a lipid (cholesterol or triglyceride) problem

eye conditions

illness of the stomach or bowel

3. You consume a lot of booze.

Before you begin taking Accutane, notify your doctor if you haven't already about any of the aforementioned.

Using different medications

If you use any additional medications, including those obtained without a prescription from a pharmacy, grocery store, or health food store, let your doctor or pharmacist know.

Accutane may be affected by certain medications. Tetracycline antibiotics, vitamin A, or medicines containing vitamin A are a few of them (including vitamin supplements)

other medications you use to treat your acne

the "mini-pill," an oral contraceptive pill that solely contains progestin.

Accutane may interact with these drugs or alter how effectively they function. You may need to take your medication in a different way or in a different dosage. You'll get advice from your doctor.

Further information about medications to be cautious of or stay away from while taking Accutane is available from your doctor and pharmacist.

If you have any questions regarding the medications on this list, see your doctor or pharmacist.

CHAPTER 2

WHAT DOSAGE TO USE

Carefully adhere to any instructions provided by your doctor or pharmacist.

These could be different from the details in this pamphlet.

Follow your doctor's instructions for taking Accutane precisely.

How many Accutane pills you should take daily will be determined by your doctor.

The dosage will be determined based on your body weight and specific demands. When your doctor learns how you react to Accutane throughout the course of therapy, this dosage may be changed.

Methods of intake

Capsules have to be consumed whole together with a glass of milk or water.

Take no broken capsules, and don't open any of the bottles.

HOW SOON TO TAKE IT

Accutane must always be taken with meals and may be taken once or twice per day.

Before beginning Accutane medication, female patients should hold off until the second or third day of their subsequent regular menstrual cycle.

By doing this, you may assist confirm that you are not pregnant before using Accutane.

Accutane should be taken as directed by your doctor.

Accutane acne therapy typically lasts 4 to 8 months. Your acne may grow a bit worse during the first few weeks of therapy before it gets better. This is not cause for concern; it shows that Accutane is having an effect.

At the conclusion of this period, your acne ought to have considerably improved. Most individuals see that their skin condition keeps getting better even after their Accutane therapy is over.

Accutane will assist in preventing future skin damage, but it cannot remove scars or pitting that existed before the start of therapy.

In case you overlook taking Accutane

Do not attempt to take an additional dosage to make up for missing ones.

The likelihood of experiencing a negative side effect might rise as a result.

If your next dosage is approaching, skip the one you missed and take the medication as scheduled.

Please let your doctor know if you've missed many doses and follow any advise they may have given you.

If you overdose on Accutane (overdose)

If you believe you or anyone else may have taken too much Accutane, call your doctor right away, the Poisons Information Center at (13 11 26), or go to Accident and Emergency at the closest hospital. Even if there are no symptoms of pain or toxicity, take this action.

You could need immediate medical care.

Overdose symptoms might include a brief headache, nausea, face flushing, red, chapped lips, stomach discomfort, headache, dizziness, and shaky gait.

Keep the phone numbers of these locations close at hand.

Throughout the course of using Accutane

Actions You Must Do

If you find out you are pregnant while using Accutane, stop taking it right away and notify your doctor.

The birth abnormalities that Accutane may cause (damage to unborn babies). You must adhere to stringent birth control measures beginning at least one month before you start taking Accutane, during treatment, and for one month after you stop.

Males who want to father children don't seem to be at danger.

Inform all healthcare providers, including your dentist, doctor, and pharmacy, that you are taking Accutane.

If for any reason you have not taken your medication precisely as directed, let your doctor know right away.

Otherwise, your doctor could assume that it wasn't successful and make an unnecessary adjustment to your therapy.

If you believe that using Accutane capsules is not improving your condition, tell your doctor.

Keep track of all of your doctor's visits so that your progress may be monitored.

Regular blood tests may be recommended by your doctor to check your liver function, blood sugar levels, and blood cholesterol levels.

Inform your doctor if you plan to undertake a lot of hard lifting or exercise.

If you engage in a lot of intense activity while taking Accutane, your muscles and joints may be more susceptible to discomfort or stiffness.

CHAPTER 3

THINGS YOU SHOULD AVOID

Without first consulting your doctor, never stop taking Accutane or adjust the dosage.

Avoid running out of medication over the weekend or during a holiday.

Despite the fact that someone else's symptoms may be identical to yours, do not give them Accutane.

Unless as directed by your doctor, do not take Accutane to treat any other conditions.

Don't give blood while using Accutane or for at least one month after quitting the medication.

ITEMS TO WATCH OUT FOR

Until you know how Accutane affects you, use caution while driving or using equipment.

Ordinarily, Accutane wouldn't impair your ability to operate equipment or drive a vehicle. Nevertheless, while using Accutane, decreased night vision and other visual abnormalities may happen. Before engaging in any activity that might be hazardous if your eyesight is impaired while taking Accutane, be sure to know how you respond to it.

Accutane therapy may make using contact lenses uncomfortable.

Dry eyes might result from rocutane. Your pharmacist may have eye lubricants or artificial tears that might help with this issue. Alternatively, you may need to wear your lenses less often or switch to wearing glasses.

When using Accutane, use sunscreen, limit your time in solariums, and avoid prolonged sun exposure.

When using Accutane, your skin can be more susceptible to sunburn.

When using Accutane and for 5 to 6 months after discontinuing Accutane therapy, avoid waxing and dermabrasion.

When using Accutane, your skin can be more sensitive. During and for many months following Accutane therapy, waxing and dermabrasion may result in scarring.

Avoid utilizing certain hair treatments, electrolysis, and face peels.

During and after your Accutane therapy, your skin and hair may be more sensitive.

CHAPTER 4

NEGATIVE EFFECTS

The majority of individuals using Accutane get relief from their acne, however some may have negative side effects.

Every medication may have unwanted consequences. Although they are sometimes severe, they are often not. If you experience any of the negative effects, you could require medical attention.

The potential adverse effects listed here should not worry you. You may not go through any of them.

Any queries you may have may be answered by your doctor or pharmacist.

If you find any of the following and they bother you, tell your doctor:

LIPS, MOUTH, NOSE, AND SKIN DRYNESS

To soften the lining of the nose, lips, and other skin regions not affected by acne, apply petroleum jelly or moisturizer.

Skin that is easily damaged changes in color and peels off on the palms and soles of the feet

itchiness on the skin and a higher risk of becoming sunburned

acne flare-ups, often at the beginning of therapy, perspiration, and changes to the nails eye issues include discharge, droopy or irritated eyes, or difficulty seeing at night

sexual dysfunction in men, including gynecomastia, diminished libido, and poor sexual function

nosebleeds

stiffness or sensitivity in your muscles, joints, or bones

tiredness \sheadache

hair fall (sometimes occurs and is usually temporary but in rare cases has persisted)

unnaturally thick hair

hoarseness

These adverse reactions are often minor and dosage dependent. If the dosage of Accutane is reduced or discontinued, the most of them vanish entirely within a few days to a few weeks.

Immediately inform your doctor if you suffer any of the following:

nausea

vomiting

ongoing headache

eyesight problems like blurriness

hearing alterations or ringing in the ears

extreme upper stomach discomfort unanticipated muscular pain, soreness, or weakness blood in the stools or severe diarrhoea severe bruises unexpected red, sometimes itchy areas beginning on the face, hands, or feet that resemble the measles rash. The spots may blister or transform into flat, circular, raised, red markings with a pale center. Moreover, you can get a fever, sore throat, headache, and/or diarrhea.

On the lips, mouth, eyes, nose, and genitals, painful red patches that progress to huge blisters and conclude with skin-layer peeling are possible. Affected individuals may have a fever, chills, achy muscles, and overall malaise.

seeing or hearing things that are not true feeling despondent, including thoughts of suicide

Feeling down or experiencing sobbing fits are among the signs of depression.

sleeping too much or having difficulties sleeping changes in your appetite or body weight losing interest in things you previously loved

having difficulty focusing

excluding yourself from your friends and family

feeling as if you lack vitality

Sense of worthlessness or excessive guilt

These negative consequences might be severe. You could need immediate medical care. Severe adverse effects are uncommon.

The list of potential adverse effects shown here is not exhaustive. Some individuals could experience others, and there might be some unidentified side effects.

Even if it's not on this list, let your doctor know if you discover anything else that is making you feel poorly.

If you don't understand anything on this list, ask your doctor or pharmacist.

Accutane Storage after use

Until you're ready to consume the capsules, keep them in the blister pack.

The capsules won't keep as well if you take them out of the container.

Accutane, like any other medication, should not be kept in a bathroom or next to a sink. Instead, keep the blister pack in a cool, dry location where the temperature is kept below 25°C.

Never leave it in the vehicle or on the sill of a window.

Certain medications may be ruined by heat and moisture.

Keep Accutane out of the reach of minors.

Medicines should be kept in a secured cabinet that is at least 1.5 meters above the ground.

Keep Accutane away from sunlight.

Ask your pharmacist how to dispose of any extra capsules if your doctor instructs you to stop taking Accutane or if the capsules are over their expiration date.

Description of the product Availability

In a box of 60 capsules, 20 mg capsules of accutane are offered.

HOW ACCUTANE APPEARS

The "ROA 20" is printed on the soft, round, half-brown-red, half-opaque white Accutane 20 mg capsule.

Ingredients Isotretinoin is the active component.

Isotretinoin 20 mg is included in each capsule of Accutane 20 mg.

The pills also include soy oil, yellow beeswax, partly hydrogenated soy oil, and hydrogenated soy oil as inactive components.

There may be residues of arachidic acid in soy oil (a component of peanut oil).

The capsule's outer shell is made of gelatin, glycerol, sorbitol, mannitol, and a substance derived from corn.

red and/or titanium dioxide iron oxide

Shellac iron oxide, a dark pigment, is included in the printing ink.

Gluten and sugar are not present in Accutane.

SUMMARY

In conclusion, Accutane is a powerful medication used to treat severe acne that has not responded to other treatments. It is highly effective in reducing the number and severity of acne lesions, and can significantly improve quality of life for individuals suffering from severe acne. However, Accutane can have potentially serious side effects and risks, including birth defects, depression, and liver damage, among others. It is important to work closely with a healthcare professional to carefully monitor dosage and duration of treatment, and to be aware of potential side effects and risks. With proper use and management, Accutane can be a valuable tool in the treatment of severe acne, but should only be used under close medical supervision.

THE END

Printed in Great Britain
by Amazon

38643467R00030